I0767759

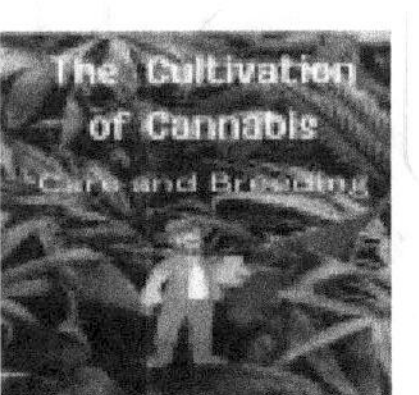
The Cultivation
of Cannabis
Care and Breeding
MARIE MORENO

Introduction about cannabis Note: Please note that the cultivation of cannabis is illegal in many countries.

Cannabis is one of the oldest crops in the world and has been used for various purposes for thousands of years. The plant has a long history as a medicine, recreational drug and as a source of textiles, paper and building materials. In recent years, cannabis has received significant attention due to its potential medicinal benefits and the growing movement for legalization for recreational use. Cannabis, also known as hemp or marijuana, comes from the Cannabaceae family and consists of three main species: Cannabis sativa, Cannabis indica and Cannabis ruderalis. The plant contains a number of chemical compounds, including more than 100 cannabinoids, the best known of which is delta-9-tetrahydrocannabinol (THC). THC is responsible for the psychoactive effects of cannabis, including the production of a euphoric 'high'. Cannabis is consumed in various forms, including smoking, vaporizing and edibles. There are also a variety of products made from cannabis, including oils, tinctures, ointments and capsules. The way cannabis is consumed affects the strength and duration of the effects, as well as the likelihood of side effects. The use of cannabis as medicine dates back thousands of years, and there is evidence that it has been used in various cultures to treat pain, nausea, cramps and other ailments. Today, there is scientific evidence that cannabis can help with a variety of conditions and symptoms, including chronic pain, multiple sclerosis, epilepsy, anxiety and nausea associated with chemotherapy. The legalization of cannabis for recreational use has gained momentum in many countries in recent years. Proponents argue that legalizing cannabis facilitates access, undermines the black market, generates tax revenue and reduces the burden on law enforcement. Opponents argue that the legalization of cannabis could lead to an increase in drug use, traffic accidents and other negative effects. In countries where cannabis has been legalized, there are various models, including legalization for recreational use, decriminalization and legalization for medical purposes. The impact of cannabis legalization is complex and can vary by country, region and circumstance. Despite the growing popularity of cannabis and efforts to push for legalization, the plant remains illegal in many countries. The illicit trade in cannabis is a lucrative business, and the illegal activities associated with cannabis can lead to violence and crime.

History of cannabis cultivation

The history of cannabis cultivation is long and varied. For thousands of years, this plant has been cultivated and used all over the world, both for medicinal and recreational purposes. The use of cannabis dates back to ancient times, where it was used in many cultures as a remedy, but also as a psychoactive drug. In this article, we will give an overview of the history of cannabis cultivation, from its beginnings to the present day. The earliest records of the use of cannabis come from China, where it has been cultivated for around 5000 years. It was used to relieve pain, reduce inflammation and treat various illnesses. Cannabis has also long been cultivated and used as a remedy in other parts of Asia, such as India and the Middle East. Over the centuries, the use of cannabis spread to other parts of the world. In the 16th century, European sailors brought the plant to North America. The English settlers in Jamestown, Virginia, used cannabis as a source of fiber to make rope and clothing. Cannabis was also cultivated and used in other parts of the world, such as Africa and South America. In the 19th century, Western scientists began to take an interest in the medicinal properties of cannabis. The Irish physician William Brooke O'Shaughnessy conducted a study in India and found that cannabis could be an effective pain treatment for rheumatism, cholera and tetanus. Cannabis was also used for medicinal purposes in Europe and North America to relieve pain, reduce anxiety and combat loss of appetite. However, in the 1920s, governments began to regulate or even ban the use of cannabis. In the US, the prohibition campaign led to the introduction of the Marihuana Tax Act in 1937, which taxed and criminalized the cultivation, sale and possession of cannabis. In the following decades, similar laws were passed in other countries. In the 1960s, however, a new movement began calling for the legalization of cannabis. This movement was driven by artists, musicians and students and spread quickly. It called for cannabis to be legalized as a recreational drug and for it to be made available for medicinal purposes. In the 1990s, medical cannabis was legalized in some states in the USA. This led to further debate about the legalization of cannabis as a recreational drug. In the decades that followed, several countries, including Canada and Uruguay, legalized or decriminalized cannabis. Other countries have legalized the use of medicinal cannabis. Today, cannabis is one of the most commonly used illegal drugs in the world.

Legality of cannabis cultivation

Cannabis cultivation is a very controversial topic and is treated differently by different countries and cultures. In some countries it is considered an illegal activity, while in others it is legalized and made available as a medical treatment. In this text, we will examine the legality of cannabis cultivation and discuss the various arguments put forward by proponents and opponents of cannabis cultivation. The legality of cannabis cultivation depends on the legislation of each country. Some countries have fully legalized the cultivation of cannabis, while others only allow cultivation for medicinal purposes and in some countries cultivation is completely prohibited. In the US, the legality of cannabis cultivation is a complex issue, as cannabis is illegal at the federal level, but many states have legalized the cultivation and sale of cannabis. Proponents of cannabis cultivation argue that cannabis is a medicinal plant and can help with various conditions, including pain, anxiety, depression, epilepsy and many other conditions. The medicinal properties of cannabis have been proven in numerous studies and there are many people who benefit from the advantages of growing cannabis. Another argument put forward by proponents of cannabis cultivation is that the legalization of cannabis cultivation would lead to decriminalization. Many people are criminalized for growing cannabis and can go to prison or pay high fines as a result. By legalizing cannabis cultivation, many people could be protected from prosecution. Opponents of cannabis cultivation, on the other hand, argue that cannabis is a gateway drug and can tempt people to try harder drugs. They also argue that growing cannabis can lead to higher crime rates, as many people may try to steal the plants or sell them illegally. Another argument against cannabis cultivation is that it can pose a risk to public health. The abuse of cannabis can lead to mental illness, and the use of cannabis can lead to accidents and injuries when people are under the influence of cannabis. Another argument against cannabis cultivation is that it can pose a danger to the environment. Cannabis cultivation requires large amounts of water and can lead to soil pollution and water consumption. In addition, the use of pesticides and fertilizers when growing cannabis can lead to environmental pollution. Overall, the legality of cannabis cultivation is a complex issue that depends on various factors. There are many arguments both for and against cannabis cultivation, and it is important to weigh all factors carefully before making a decision.

Benefits and risks of cannabis cultivation

Cannabis cultivation is a topic that has long been the subject of controversy. In some countries, cannabis cultivation is legal, while in others it is illegal. There are numerous benefits and risks of cannabis cultivation, which are explained below. Benefits of cannabis cultivation Medical use: One of the most well-known medical uses of cannabis is to relieve pain in cancer patients. Cannabis can also help in the treatment of epilepsy, nausea and anxiety. Some studies have also shown that cannabis can be helpful in the treatment of Alzheimer's disease and Parkinson's disease. Economic benefits: Legal cannabis cultivation can lead to economic benefits as it creates jobs and generates tax revenue. In some countries where cannabis cultivation is legal, legalization has led to an increase in tourism. Environmental benefits: Cannabis is a plant that grows quickly and absorbs carbon dioxide. Therefore, growing cannabis can help to reduce carbon levels in the atmosphere. Cultural significance: Cannabis has a long history of cultural significance and is considered a sacred plant by many people. Growing cannabis can help to preserve and promote this cultural significance. Risks of cannabis cultivation Health risks: The use of cannabis can lead to health risks, especially when consumed in large quantities and over a long period of time. Cannabis can lead to memory loss, confusion, anxiety and paranoia. Criminal activity: Illegal cannabis cultivation can lead to criminal activity, such as selling cannabis on the black market. This can lead to violence and other forms of crime. Environmental pollution: The cultivation of cannabis can lead to environmental pollution, especially if the cultivation is done with chemical fertilizers and pesticides. These chemicals can leach into groundwater and other bodies of water and damage the environment. Addiction: Cannabis can be addictive, especially when consumed in large quantities and over a long period of time. Addiction to cannabis can lead to health problems and social problems. Protection of minors: The cultivation of cannabis can lead to young people having easier access to cannabis, especially if cultivation is not regulated. This can lead to an increase in the use of cannabis by young people. Conclusion Cannabis cultivation has both benefits and risks. The medicinal applications of cannabis can help to alleviate illnesses and improve the well-being of patients.

Choosing the right cannabis strain

Choosing the right cannabis strain can be a challenge, as there are a variety of strains that differ in their effects and flavor. Before deciding on a strain, it is important to understand the effects and properties you expect from using cannabis. There are three main types of cannabis strains: sativa, indica and hybrid. Each strain has its own characteristics that are suitable for different purposes. Sativa strains are often described as energizing and euphoric. They are ideal for daytime use or outdoor activities. Sativas can also help to increase creativity and improve focus. The plants are usually taller and have thin leaves. The flowering time of sativa strains is longer than indica strains and can be up to 14 weeks. Indica strains are often described as relaxing and calming. They are well suited for use in the evening or before bedtime. Indicas can also help to relieve pain and anxiety. The plants are usually smaller and have wider leaves. The flowering time of indica strains is shorter than sativa strains and is usually 8-12 weeks. Hybrid strains are a mixture of sativa and indica strains. The effects of hybrid strains can vary depending on the composition of the strains. Some hybrids can be energizing and help improve focus, while others can be calming and relaxing. The flowering time of hybrids can vary depending on the composition of the strains. When choosing a cannabis strain, it's important to consider THC and CBD levels. THC is the psychoactive component of cannabis and is responsible for the 'high' effect, while CBD is responsible for the medicinal benefits of cannabis. Sativa strains often have higher THC levels than indica strains, while indica strains can have higher CBD levels. For medicinal purposes, strains with higher CBD levels may be preferred, as CBD is known for its anti-inflammatory and pain-relieving properties. For recreational purposes, strains with higher THC levels may be preferred as they have a more intense effect. Another important factor when choosing a cannabis strain is the taste. Each strain has its own unique taste and smell. Some strains have fruity or floral aromas, while others have earthy or spicy notes. It is important to choose a strain that suits individual taste preferences to ensure the best possible experience.

Growing conditions for cannabis

Cannabis is a plant that needs to grow under certain conditions to reach its maximum size and potential. In this article, we will discuss the most important factors that influence cannabis growth. Light Light is a crucial factor for the growth of cannabis. If cannabis plants do not receive enough light, they grow slowly and remain small. The ideal amount of light for cannabis is between 600 and 1000 micromoles per second. It is important that the plants receive at least 18 hours of light per day during the vegetation phase and at least 12 hours of darkness per day during the flowering phase. Humidity Humidity also plays an important role in the growth of cannabis. If the humidity is too high, mold can form, which impairs growth and increases the risk of disease. The ideal humidity level is between 40% and 60%. During the vegetation phase, cannabis plants require a higher humidity than during the flowering phase. Temperature Temperature is another important factor for the growth of cannabis. The ideal temperature is between 20°C and 28°C. If the temperature is too high, the plants can dry out and burn. If the temperature is too low, this can slow down growth and increase the risk of disease. Air circulation Good air circulation is important to promote the growth of cannabis. Good ventilation ensures that the plants receive enough CO2 and that the humidity is controlled. It is also important to ensure that the air circulation does not dry out the plants too much or make them too cold. Soil and nutrients The choice of soil and the nutrients supplied to the plant are also important factors in the growth of cannabis. A good soil should have adequate drainage to ensure that water does not remain in the soil and rot the roots. The soil should also contain enough nutrients to support the plant's growth. It is advisable to use fertilizers with a high nitrogen content during the vegetation phase and fertilizers with a high phosphorus content during the flowering phase. pH value The pH value of the soil is another important factor for the growth of cannabis. The ideal pH value is between 6 and 7. If the pH value is too high or too low, the plants cannot absorb nutrients properly and growth is impaired. It is important to monitor the pH value regularly and adjust it if necessary. Plant care Good plant care is also important to ensure the growth of cannabis !!!!!!

Cultivation systems for cannabis

Cannabis cultivation is a topic that has received more and more attention in recent years. The legalization of cannabis in some countries has led to more and more people wanting to grow their own cannabis. There are different growing systems for cannabis that can be chosen depending on the needs of the grower and the conditions of the grow. In this article, we will take a closer look at some of the most important cannabis cultivation systems. Indoor cultivation Growing cannabis indoors is one of the most common methods. This method is particularly suitable for people who live in areas where growing cannabis is illegal or for those who want to grow cannabis all year round. With indoor cultivation, the cannabis is grown in an enclosed space where all parameters such as light, temperature, humidity and airflow can be controlled by the grower.

It is also possible to use different growing systems for indoor cultivation, such as hydroponics, aeroponics or traditional soil. Outdoor cultivation Outdoor cannabis cultivation is the oldest and most natural method of growing cannabis. This method is particularly suitable for people who have enough outdoor space to grow cannabis, as well as for those who want to grow cannabis in a sustainable and environmentally friendly way. When growing outdoors, it is important that the cannabis is grown in an area with sufficient sunlight and good soil quality. It is also important to protect the cannabis from pests and diseases by pruning and treating it regularly. Greenhouse cultivation The greenhouse cultivation of cannabis is a mixture of indoor and outdoor cultivation. This method is particularly suitable for people who want the benefits of indoor growing but also appreciate the natural environment of outdoor growing. In greenhouse cultivation, the cannabis is grown in an enclosed space where all parameters such as light, temperature, humidity and airflow can be controlled by the grower. It is also possible to use different growing systems for greenhouse cultivation, such as hydroponics, aeroponics or traditional soil. Hydroponic cultivation Hydroponic cultivation of cannabis is a method in which the cannabis is grown in a nutrient solution rather than in traditional soil. This method is particularly suitable for people who want to maximize the yield and speed of cultivation. In hydroponic growing, the cannabis is grown in an enclosed space where all parameters such as light, temperature, humidity and airflow can be controlled by the grower. It is also possible to use different types of hydroponic systems, such as Deep Water Culture (DWC), Ebb and Flow or NFT (Nutrient Film Technique). Aeroponic cannabis cultivation is a method where the cannabis is grown in the air rather than in traditional soil.

Indoor cannabis cultivation

Indoor cannabis cultivation has gained popularity in recent years as a way to control and optimize the growth of cannabis plants. In this article, we will focus on growing cannabis indoors and discuss everything you need to know to successfully run your own facility. Preparing the space Before you start growing cannabis indoors, you need to prepare the space where the plants will grow. First, you need to clean and sanitize the space to ensure that there are no fungi or bacteria that could affect the growth of your plants. Next, you need to make sure that the room is sufficiently ventilated. To do this, you can install an exhaust system or a fan to circulate the air and reduce humidity. The humidity in the room should be between 40 and 60% to ensure optimal growth. Finally, you need to make sure that the room is adequately lit. You can use LED lamps or sodium vapor lamps to optimize the light spectrum and promote the growth of your plants. Choosing the right strain When choosing the right strain for growing cannabis indoors, make sure you choose a strain that is suitable for indoor growing. Some strains are better suited to outdoor cultivation, while others are better suited to indoor cultivation. In addition, you should also consider the type of effect you want to achieve when selecting the variety. Some varieties are better suited for medicinal use, while others are more suitable for recreational use. Germinating and growing the plants Once you have chosen the right strain, you can start germinating and growing your plants. For this you will need high-quality seeds and a germination table or germination bag. Once the seeds have germinated, you can report them in pots or grow boxes. It is important that you water and fertilize the plants regularly to ensure optimal growth. You should also ensure that the temperature and humidity in the room remain constant to promote healthy growth. Vegetation and flowering phase The vegetation phase is the time when your plants are growing and developing. During this time, you should ensure that your plants receive enough light, water and nutrients. It is also important that you prune the plants regularly to promote growth and improve air circulation. The flowering phase is the time when your plants develop flowers and mature.

Growing cannabis outdoors

Growing cannabis outdoors, also known as outdoor cultivation, is one way to produce high-quality cannabis. In outdoor cultivation, the plant is grown in natural conditions, which usually results in larger plants with higher yields. Below are some important factors to consider when growing cannabis outdoors. Location and climate Choosing the right location for growing cannabis is crucial. Cannabis needs plenty of sunlight to grow and thrive properly. For this reason, the growing location should be chosen so that the plants have the greatest possible access to sunlight. Ideally, the growing location should be fully exposed to sunlight and have no obstructions such as trees or buildings that hinder access to sunlight. Climate is another important factor to consider. Cannabis grows best at temperatures between 18 and 30 degrees Celsius. Temperatures that are too high or too low can affect the growth and development of the plants. If the growing location is in a region with a humid climate, this can lead to mold growth on the plants, which can affect the harvest. Soil and fertilization Soil is another important factor when growing cannabis outdoors. The soil should be rich in nutrients to support the growth of the plants. One way to ensure that the soil contains enough nutrients is to use organic fertilizers. The use of chemical fertilizers can affect soil life and leave unwanted chemical residues in the cannabis. Irrigation Irrigation is another important factor when growing cannabis outdoors. Cannabis requires regular watering to grow and develop. In general, cannabis plants need about 3-4 liters of water per day. If the growing location is in a region with high humidity, it is particularly important to ensure that the plants do not get too wet, as this can lead to mold growth. Pest control is a challenge when growing cannabis outdoors. There are many types of pests that can infest cannabis plants, such as aphids, spider mites and thrips. One way to repel pests is to use natural insecticides such as neem oil. Another option is to use predators such as ladybugs and spiders that eat pests, thus minimizing the use of chemicals. Harvesting and drying Harvesting and drying are the final steps in outdoor cannabis cultivation. The plants should be Hydroponic cultivation of cannabis The hydroponic cultivation of cannabis has become increasingly important in recent years. In contrast to traditional soil cultivation, this method allows greater control over nutrient uptake and plant growth. In this article, we will take a closer look at hydroponic cannabis cultivation and examine the advantages and disadvantages as well as the different methods and systems.

Hydroponic cannabis cultivation - what is it?

Hydroponic cultivation refers to growing plants without soil. Instead, the roots are kept in a water- and nutrient-rich medium such as rockwool, coconut fibers, perlite or vermiculite. The advantage of this method is that the grower has complete control over the nutrient uptake and growth of the plant. This means that you can precisely dose which nutrients and how much water the plant receives. This can lead to higher yields and better plants. Advantages and disadvantages of hydroponic cannabis cultivation Advantages: Faster growth: By providing the plant with an optimal supply of nutrients and water, it can grow faster. Higher yields: When all factors are controlled, yields can be higher compared to traditional soil cultivation. Less space required: As the plants grow in a medium instead of in the soil, the space required can be reduced. Less chance of pest infestation: As the soil is no longer a potential source of pests and diseases, there is less chance of pest infestation. Reduced risk of soil contamination: There can be an accumulation of contaminants in the soil that can affect the plant. Hydroponic cultivation eliminates this risk. Disadvantages: Higher costs: setting up a hydroponic grow can be expensive as you may need specialized equipment and materials. More effort: Hydroponic cultivation requires more effort and knowledge than traditional soil cultivation. You need to regularly monitor the pH of the water and adjust the nutrient content of the medium. Less flexible: Once you have set up a hydroponic system, it is more difficult to change or move it. Hydroponic growing methods for cannabis There are various hydroponic growing methods for cannabis, which we will now look at in more detail. Deep Water Culture (DWC) DWC is one of the simplest hydroponic growing methods. The plants are placed in a container with water and nutrients, which is illuminated from below. The roots hang in the water and absorb the nutrients. DWC systems are relatively inexpensive.

Aeroponic cultivation of cannabis

Aeroponic cannabis cultivation is a method of growing cannabis in which plants are grown in an airy environment and receive their nutrients in the form of fine mist droplets. Unlike other growing methods, such as hydroponics or soil cultivation, the aeroponic method requires less water and offers greater control over the plants' growth. In this article, we will discuss the advantages and disadvantages of growing cannabis aeroponically. The benefits of growing cannabis aeroponically Higher yields Growing cannabis aeroponically can result in higher yields than other growing methods. This is because the roots of the plants are kept in a moist, nutrient-rich environment that encourages their growth. The plants can also be planted at a closer spacing, resulting in a higher yield per square meter. Fewer pest problems As the plants are suspended in the air and their roots remain in a closed container, they are less susceptible to pest infestation. Pests that normally attack the soil or plant surface cannot reach the roots, reducing the risk of infection. Less water and nutrients required Aeroponic cannabis cultivation requires less water and nutrients compared to other cultivation methods. This is because the nutrient solution is sprayed directly onto the roots of the plants, making the use of water and nutrients more efficient. This can also reduce the amount of waste and waste water. Faster growth As the roots of the plants are kept in a moist environment, they can grow and spread quickly. The plants are able to absorb more nutrients, which leads to faster growth. This can shorten the cultivation time. The disadvantages of growing cannabis aeroponically High costs The initial costs for an aeroponic system are higher than for other cultivation methods. Special containers, pumps, nozzles and sensors need to be purchased to spray the nutrient solution and monitor the environment. This can be a challenge for the beginner or hobby gardener. High air quality requirements Air quality is an important factor for successful aeroponic cultivation. The environment must be clean and free of contaminants that could affect the health of the plants. The room must also be well ventilated to ensure air circulation.

Soil and nutrients for cannabis

Soil and nutrients are crucial for the growth and development of cannabis. Proper care and management of the soil and nutrients is necessary to obtain a healthy plant with high quality. In this article, we will look at the main factors necessary for the growth of cannabis, including the soil, nutrients and key ingredients necessary for the growth and development of the plant. The soil Choosing the right soil is an important factor in growing cannabis. There are different types of soil, but the most suitable soil for cannabis is a slightly acidic, loose and nutrient-rich soil with a pH between 6 and 7. A well-drained soil is important so that the plant's roots receive enough oxygen and water can drain away easily. Soil with too much moisture can damage the roots and encourage mold growth. Soil with too little water can inhibit the plant's growth and lead to a lack of nutrients. To ensure that the soil is sufficiently rich in nutrients, fertilizer can be added. The fertilizer should contain nitrogen, phosphorus and potassium, which are the most important nutrients for cannabis growth. However, it is important that the fertilizer is not overdosed, as this can damage the plant. Too high a concentration of nutrients can lead to nutrient burn and damage the roots. It is also important to ensure that the fertilizer is not too acidic, as this can change the pH value of the soil and thus impair the growth of the plant. Nutrients Nutrients are crucial for the growth of cannabis. The most important nutrients are nitrogen, phosphorus and potassium. Nitrogen is necessary for the growth of the leaves and the stem of the plant. Phosphorus is important for the development of the plant's roots, flowers and fruits. Potassium promotes growth and increases the plant's resistance to pests and diseases. There are different types of fertilizers that can be used for cannabis. Organic fertilizers are a natural alternative to chemical fertilizers and can be made from animal manure, compost or other organic materials. Organic fertilizers often contain a variety of nutrients that are more easily absorbed by the plant, while also promoting the growth of beneficial microorganisms in the soil. However, chemical fertilizers can also be very effective as long as they are correctly dosed and applied. pH and EC in cannabis cultivation pH and EC are important parameters to consider when growing cannabis. The pH value indicates how acidic or alkaline a solution is, while the EC value measures the conductivity of a solution. Both values can have a significant impact on the growth and health of cannabis. pH value in cannabis cultivation: The pH value plays a crucial role in cannabis cultivation as it affects the availability of nutrients. Most nutrients are best available in a pH range of 5.5 to 6.5. If the pH is too high or too low, the plants cannot grow and thrive optimally. A pH of 7 or higher can cause nutrients such as iron and manganese to become unavailable, while a pH below 5 can affect the absorption of calcium and magnesium. A pH value that is too high or too low can also make plants more susceptible to diseases and pests. Fungal diseases such as Fusarium and Pythium are more common when the pH is too high, while spider mites and thrips are more common when the pH is low. It is therefore important to monitor the pH regularly and take appropriate measures to ensure that it remains within the optimal range. EC value in cannabis cultivation: The EC value is a measure of the conductivity of a solution and indicates how many dissolved salts are in the solution. In cannabis cultivation, it is important to monitor the EC value of the nutrient mixture to ensure that the plants receive the right amount of nutrients. Too high an EC level can cause the plants to suffer burns and other damage, while too low an EC level can lead to a lack of nutrients. It is important to measure the EC value regularly and make appropriate adjustments to ensure that the plants receive the right amount of nutrients. An EC value that is too high can be lowered by rinsing the plants with clear water, while an EC value that is too low can be increased by adding nutrients. Monitoring pH and EC in cannabis cultivation: Monitoring pH and EC levels when growing cannabis is an important step in ensuring that plants grow and thrive optimally. There are several ways to measure pH and EC, including the use of pH and EC meters. pH meters are usually quite accurate and can be easy to use.

Light requirements and light cycles in cannabis cultivation

Light is one of the most important elements for the growth and development of plants, including cannabis. The quality, intensity and duration of light directly affect the cannabis growth process and can have a significant impact on yields and the quality of the end products. Light requirements: of cannabis Cannabis is a plant that requires high light intensity to grow and develop optimally. In nature, cannabis usually grows in tropical or subtropical regions where the sunlight is intense and the climate is warm and humid. When cannabis is grown indoors, the plants' : light requirements must be met by artificial light sources. In general, it is recommended to use at least 400-600 watts of artificial light per square meter to meet the light requirements of cannabis during the growth and flowering phase. It is also important to consider the color of the light used to grow cannabis. Plants need light in the blue and red spectrum to grow optimally. During the vegetative phase of the cannabis plant, the light spectrum should emphasize more blue, while more red light is preferred during the flowering phase. Light cycles in cannabis cultivation Another important factor for cannabis cultivation is the light cycle. Cannabis is a photoperiodic plant, which means that its flowering is influenced by the duration of the light and dark cycle. Most strains of cannabis require a dark period of 12 hours per day to enter the flowering phase. During the vegetative phase of the cannabis plant, a light cycle of 18 hours of light and 6 hours of darkness is usually recommended. This ratio of light and darkness helps the plant to optimize its metabolic processes and promote growth. Once the cannabis plant is ready to enter the flowering phase, the light cycle should be switched to 12 hours of light and 12 hours of darkness. This ratio of light and dark helps the plant to go into flowering and produce flowers. It is important to maintain the light cycle consistently during the flowering stage of the cannabis plant, as interrupting the light cycle can cause a delay in flowering and yields can be reduced. Final thoughts Overall, light is one of the most important factors for cannabis cultivation and can have a significant impact on the quality and quantity of the end products.

It is important to understand the light requirements of cannabis and ensure that plants receive sufficient light to grow optimally.

Temperature and humidity conditions in cannabis cultivation

When growing cannabis, it is of great importance to carefully control and monitor the temperature and humidity conditions. If these conditions are not optimal, this can lead to a poorer quality crop and increased susceptibility to pest infestation and disease. This article explains the ideal temperature and humidity conditions for cannabis cultivation and the effects of deviations from these conditions. Temperature conditions Temperature conditions for cannabis cultivation are important as they affect the growth, development and quality of the harvest. The ideal temperature for cannabis cultivation is between 21 and 29 degrees Celsius during the vegetative phase. During the flowering phase, the temperature should be kept at around 18 to 26 degrees Celsius. It is important to note that the temperature difference between day and night should not be more than 6 degrees Celsius. Excessively high temperatures can lead to heat stress, which can inhibit plant growth and affect the quality of the harvest. If the temperatures are too high, the leaves and flowers of the plants can dry out and curl. This can also lead to increased susceptibility to pests and diseases. It is important to use air conditioning and fans to keep the temperature at an appropriate level. Too low temperatures can also affect the growth and quality of the crop. If temperatures are too low, the plants may grow more slowly and remain smaller. This can also lead to increased susceptibility to pests and diseases. It is important to use heaters to keep the temperature at an appropriate level. Humidity conditions Humidity conditions for cannabis cultivation are also important as they affect the growth, development and quality of the harvest. The ideal relative humidity (RH) during the vegetative phase is between 40 and 70 percent. During the flowering phase, the relative humidity should be kept at around 40 to 50 percent. Excessive humidity can lead to problems, as this encourages the growth of mold and bacteria. Mold can infect the plants and flowers and cause them to become inedible. If the humidity is too high, this can also lead to increased susceptibility to pests. It is important to use dehumidifiers to keep the humidity at an appropriate level. Too low humidity can also lead to problems, as this can inhibit plant growth. If the humidity is too low, the leaves of the plants can dry out.

Air circulation and CO2 supply in cannabis cultivation

Air circulation and CO2 supply are decisive factors in successful cannabis cultivation. Optimal air circulation and CO2 supply help to ensure that the plants grow healthily and a maximum harvest is achieved. Air circulation in cannabis cultivation Good air circulation is important for successful cannabis cultivation. The plants need fresh air to breathe and absorb the CO2 they need to grow. Poor air circulation can lead to a build-up of moisture, which encourages the growth of mold and other fungi. Poor air circulation can also cause pests such as spider mites and thrips to colonize the plant. Good air circulation can be achieved by using fans. The fans should be positioned so that they distribute the air evenly throughout the room. Ideally, the air in a cannabis plant should be completely exchanged every 1-2 minutes. This can be achieved by using vents or an exhaust system. Temperature and humidity also play an important role in air circulation. The temperature should be between 21°C and 26°C and the humidity should be between 40% and 60%. Humidity that is too high can lead to mold growth, while humidity that is too low can impair plant growth. CO2 supply in cannabis cultivation CO2 is an essential component for the growth of plants. A sufficient CO2 supply can lead to a higher harvest and a faster growth rate. As a rule, the air contains around 400 ppm (parts per million) CO2. A higher CO2 content in the air can accelerate the growth of plants and increase crop yields. There are several ways to increase the CO2 supply in a cannabis plant. One option is to use CO2 generators that release CO2 into the room. Another option is to use CO2 tanks that release the gas directly into the room. However, both options require close monitoring of the CO2 level in the air to ensure that it does not get too high and harm the plants. An alternative method of supplying CO2 is to use plant extracts that are rich in CO2. For example, fermented plant material or compost tea can be used to increase CO2 levels. However, this method is less accurate than using CO2 generators or tanks. Conclusion Good air circulation and CO2 supply are crucial factors for successful cannabis cultivation.

Pest control in cannabis cultivation

Pest control in cannabis cultivation is a decisive factor for a successful harvest. Pests can impair plant growth, reduce yields and even affect the quality of the flowers. There are a variety of pests that can be encountered when growing cannabis, including spider mites, aphids, thrips, whiteflies and caterpillars. In this article, various methods of pest control are presented. Biological pest control Biological pest control can be an effective method of controlling pests in cannabis cultivation. Natural enemies of the pests are used to decimate them. This method is environmentally friendly and can promote plant health. The most common natural enemies of pests are beneficial insects such as ladybugs, predatory mites, parasitic wasps and lacewings. However, the use of beneficial insects requires careful planning and implementation. It is important to select the right beneficial insects to ensure that they control the pest causing the problem. In addition, the conditions in the growing environment must be right to ensure that the beneficial insects feel comfortable and can do their job. Chemical pest control Chemical pest control is another method of controlling pests in cannabis cultivation. It is important to choose the right chemicals to ensure that they effectively control the pests without harming the plants. There are many chemical pesticides on the market, but not all of them are suitable for use in cannabis cultivation. It is important to follow the manufacturer's instructions and only use the chemicals at the recommended dosage. Some of the most common pesticides used in cannabis cultivation are pyrethroids, neonicotinoids and organophosphates. Pyrethroids are synthetic chemicals derived from chrysanthemum flowers. They are often used to control spider mites and whiteflies. Neonicotinoids are chemicals that attack the nervous system of insects and are often used to control aphids and thrips. Organophosphates are chemicals that attack the nervous system of pests and are often used to control caterpillars. However, it is important to point out that chemical pesticides are not without risks. They can kill not only the pests, but also beneficial insects and pollute the environment.

Disease control in cannabis cultivation

Growing cannabis can be a difficult task for some people, especially when it comes to dealing with disease. There are many factors that can lead to disease in cannabis plants, such as pests, fungal infestations, deficiencies and environmental factors. Fortunately, there are a variety of methods to combat diseases in cannabis cultivation. One of the most effective ways to combat disease in cannabis cultivation is prevention. It is important that cannabis plants are grown in a clean environment and that humidity and temperature are controlled to prevent the growth of mold and other pathogens. Regularly removing wilted leaves and unwanted material from the grow room can help minimize the risk of disease. Another important way to prevent disease in cannabis plants is to choose more resistant strains. There are many strains of cannabis that are resistant to mold and other pathogens. By choosing such varieties, you can significantly reduce the risk of diseases in cannabis cultivation. However, if a disease develops in the cannabis grow despite all precautions, it is important to act quickly to prevent the spread. One way to do this is to use biological pesticides and fungicides that can naturally fight pathogens without harming the plant itself. Examples of such biological products are Bacillus thuringiensis and Trichoderma. If biological pesticides and fungicides are not enough to control a disease in cannabis cultivation, there are also chemical pesticides and fungicides that can be used. However, it is important to be careful when using chemical products and ensure that they are suitable for use in cannabis cultivation. Chemical pesticides and fungicides can be toxic and should therefore only be used to a limited extent. In addition to the use of pesticides and fungicides, there are other methods of disease control in cannabis cultivation. One option is the use of beneficial insects such as ladybugs and predatory mites, which can eat pests and pathogens. Another method is to use water and air sterilization systems to prevent the spread of pathogens. Deficiencies can also lead to disease in cannabis plants. Monitoring nutrient deficiencies and properly fertilizing plants can help prevent deficiencies and promote plant growth. It is also important to ensure that cannabis plants are not overwatered.

Harvest time and harvesting methods for cannabis

Cannabis is a plant that has been known for centuries for its medicinal and psychoactive properties. In recent years, the legalization of cannabis has led to an increase in demand for cannabis products in many parts of the world. However, the cultivation of cannabis requires special attention, especially in terms of harvest time and harvesting methods, to ensure that the plant reaches its maximum potency and the quality of the harvest is guaranteed. The harvest time of cannabis is crucial as it affects the quality and potency of the crop. The time of harvest depends on the type of cannabis plant, the strain, the growth cycle and the growing conditions. A general rule is that cannabis should be harvested when the trichomes on the flowers have fully developed. Trichomes are the resinous crystals on the flowers that contain the cannabinoids responsible for the medicinal and psychoactive effects of cannabis. They can be easily visualized with a microscope as they look like small, shiny crystals. If the trichomes are milky white or amber in color, this is an indication that the cannabinoids have reached their peak and the plant is ready to be harvested. Another way to determine when to harvest is to observe the color of the pistils. The pistils are small hairs that grow from the flowers, and they will be white during the growth cycle. However, as they near the end of the growth cycle, they will change from white to an orange or reddish color. When most of the pistils of a flower have changed color, this is another sign that the plant is ready to be harvested. Overall, the harvest time of cannabis is a critical factor that affects the quality and potency of the crop. Harvesting too early or too late can affect the quality and potency of the crop, potentially resulting in a lower yield. Harvesting methods There are various harvesting methods that can be used when harvesting cannabis. The harvesting method usually depends on the size of the growing area, the type of cannabis plant and the equipment available. Below are some of the most common harvesting methods. Hand harvesting: With hand harvesting, each plant is harvested individually. This method works well for smaller grow spaces and allows the grower to look at each plant individually to ensure it is fully mature.

Drying and curing cannabis

Cannabis is a plant known for its psychoactive compounds, particularly tetrahydrocannabinol (THC) and cannabidiol (CBD). In many countries, cannabis is being legalized for medical and/or recreational purposes, and there is a growing demand for high-quality cannabis. Drying and curing are crucial steps in the processing of cannabis to improve the quality, flavor and aroma and to ensure that the final product is safe and long-lasting. This article takes a closer look at the drying and curing of cannabis. Drying cannabis After harvesting, cannabis flowers need to be dried to remove excess moisture and activate the active ingredients. Too much moisture can cause mold to form and render the end product unusable. The optimum moisture content for dried cannabis is around 10-15%. Drying can be done in a variety of ways, but the most common approach is to hang the cannabis flowers upside down and store them in a dark, ventilated place. The ideal temperature for drying cannabis is between 18 and 24 degrees Celsius. During the drying process, the flowers should be checked regularly to ensure that they do not dry too quickly or remain moist for too long. Another method of drying is the use of drying devices. These devices use airflow and/or heat to remove moisture from the cannabis flowers. While this method can be faster, it can also affect the quality of the final product if not done correctly. Curing cannabis After drying, the cannabis must undergo a curing process to develop the full aroma, flavor and effect. Curing is a slow process in which the moisture inside the cannabis flowers is evenly distributed and the carboxylic acid form of THC is converted into the active psychoactive form. For curing, the cannabis flowers are stored in airtight containers. During curing, the container should be opened daily to release excess moisture and allow fresh air to enter. The ideal humidity for curing cannabis is between 55 and 62%. If the humidity is too high, mold and rot can occur, while too low humidity can affect the aroma and taste. The duration of curing can vary depending on the characteristics of the cannabis and the conditions, but generally it takes 2-6 weeks. During curing, the color and aroma may change.

Processing cannabis flowers into smoking products

Cannabis flowers are the most common form of cannabis consumed. The flowers contain psychoactive compounds known as cannabinoids. These compounds can be consumed in a variety of ways, including smoking. This article describes the steps involved in processing cannabis flowers into smoking products. Step 1: Drying the cannabis flowers The first step in processing cannabis flowers into smoking products is to dry them. This process allows the moisture to be removed from the flowers to provide a better smoking experience. If cannabis flowers are too moist, they cannot burn properly and smoking becomes difficult. Drying can be done by hanging the flowers in a dark and ventilated place until they are completely dry. Step 2: Removal of stems and seeds After drying, the cannabis flowers must be freed from stems and seeds. Stems and seeds affect the smoking experience and can negatively influence the taste and effect of the product. It is important to go through the flowers thoroughly to ensure that all stems and seeds are removed. Step 3: Crushing the cannabis flowers Once the cannabis flowers have been dried and the stems and seeds have been removed, they need to be crushed. This can be done with a grinder or by hand. Crushing the flowers increases the surface area, which improves the smoking experience and makes it easier to absorb the active ingredients. Step 4: Choosing the smoking device There are different types of smoking devices that can be used to smoke cannabis flowers. Among the most popular are pipes, bongs, joints and vaporizers. It is important to choose the right smoking device to ensure an optimal smoking experience. Each method has its pros and cons, but ultimately it comes down to personal preference as to which device is most suitable. Step 5: Filling the smoking device Once the smoking device has been selected, the cannabis flowers must be filled into the device. The amount of flowers depends on the size of the smoking device and the desired effect. It is important not to fill too much at once to avoid overloading and to ensure an optimal smoking experience. Step 6: Lighting the cannabis flowers Once the smoking device is filled with cannabis flowers, it needs to be lit. Care must be taken here to avoid injury. It is important to hold the device securely and not place the fire too close to your face.

Processing cannabis flowers in to edibles

Cannabis is increasingly being used for its medicinal and recreational properties, and many people prefer to consume it in edible form. However, processing cannabis flowers into edibles requires a certain amount of knowledge and caution to ensure a safe and effective dose. In this article, we'll look at processing cannabis flower into edibles and share some tips and tricks to get the most out of your cannabis treats. Before processing cannabis flower into edibles, it's important to understand the differences between smoking cannabis and eating cannabis. When cannabis is smoked, the THC goes directly into the lungs and then into the blood, which can lead to a quick and intense high. In contrast, when cannabis is eaten, it has to pass through the digestive tract before entering the bloodstream. This can lead to a delayed and longer-lasting effect, which can last up to 6 hours. It is therefore important to dose correctly to avoid an overdose. The first step in processing cannabis flowers into edibles is to decarboxylate the flowers. This means that they need to be heated to convert the inactive THCA into active THC. Without this step, the THC will not be able to release its psychoactive effects. To decarboxylate the flowers, they can be heated in a preheated pan or oven at 110-120 degrees Celsius for around 30-45 minutes. This activates the THC and makes the flowers ready for further processing. After decarboxylation, the flowers can be processed into a variety of edibles, such as brownies, cookies, gummy bears or even pizza. However, the easiest way to incorporate cannabis flowers into edibles is through the production of cannabutter or cannaoil. This is done by mixing the decarboxylated cannabis flower with butter or oil and then melting it in a pot over low heat. The mixture is heated for around 2-3 hours and stirred regularly to ensure that the THC is evenly distributed. Once cooked, the mixture can be filtered through a sieve to remove the plant materials, and the finished cannabutter or cannaoil can be used for a variety of recipes. However, it is important to measure the dosage of cannabutter or cannaoil accurately to avoid overdosing. Too high a dose can lead to an unpleasant high that can last for several hours. A good rule of thumb is to start with a low dose and then slowly increase until the desired effect occurs.

Manufacturing of cannabis extracts and concentrations

The production of cannabis extracts and concentrates is an important part of the cannabis industry. There are many different methods of extracting cannabinoids from the cannabis plant, each with their own advantages and disadvantages. In this article, we will take a closer look at the different methods of producing cannabis extracts and concentrations, as well as their pros and cons. The most common methods of extracting cannabinoids from the cannabis plant are solvent extraction, CO_2 extraction, alcohol extraction and water extraction. Each method has its own advantages and disadvantages and is more suitable for certain applications than others. Solvent extraction is one of the oldest methods of producing cannabis extracts and concentrations. This method uses a liquid solvent such as butane, ethanol or isopropyl alcohol to extract the cannabinoids from the plant. The extraction process can be carried out either by immersing the plant materials in the solvent or by using pressure and heat. The extracted solution is then vaporized to remove the solvent and obtain a concentrated extract. Solvent extraction is a fast and efficient method of extracting large amounts of cannabinoids. However, the solvent can leave residues in the extract that can be potentially toxic. Therefore, such extracts must be carefully tested and purified before they can be commercialized. Solvent extraction is most commonly used for the production of oils, waxes and resins. CO_2

extraction is one of the most modern and advanced methods for producing cannabis extracts and concentrations. In this method, carbon dioxide is used at high pressure and low temperature to extract the cannabinoids from the plant. The CO_2 is passed through the plant, extracting the cannabinoids and collecting them as a liquid concentrate. CO_2 extraction is a very precise method that allows a high level of control over the extraction process. It can also be used to produce different types of cannabis extracts such as oils, waxes, resins and even isolates. However, the disadvantage of this method is that it is more expensive than solvent extraction. Alcohol extraction is another commonly used method for producing cannabis extracts and concentrations. This method uses alcohol as a solvent to extract the cannabinoids from the plant. It is also one of the safest methods of extracting cannabinoids, as alcohol is a non-toxic solvent that evaporates easily and leaves no residue.

Extraction of cannabinoids from cannabis

Cannabinoid extraction from cannabis is an important step in the production of medical or recreational cannabis products. The cannabis plant contains over 100 cannabinoids, the best known of which are tetrahydrocannabinol (THC) and cannabidiol (CBD). Other important cannabinoids are cannabinol (CBN), cannabigerol (CBG) and cannabichromene (CBC). Extraction of cannabinoids from cannabis can be done in several ways, and the choice of method depends on various factors, such as the desired cannabinoid composition, the size of the production batch and the available resources. One of the oldest and simplest methods of cannabinoid extraction is the production of cannabis oil using a carrier oil such as olive oil or coconut oil. This method is known as the "maceration method". The method is simple and does not require expensive equipment, but the yield of cannabinoids is usually low. Another method of extracting cannabinoids from cannabis is the use of solvents. This involves making a solution of a solvent and the cannabinoids, which is then separated from the plant materials by filtration or distillation. A well-known solvent for this method is ethanol. Another method for extracting cannabinoids from cannabis is the use of supercritical CO2 (carbon dioxide). This method is particularly popular as it allows for a high yield of cannabinoids and is considered safe and effective. The process uses CO2 under high pressure and high temperatures to extract the desired cannabinoid from the plant. The carbon dioxide serves as a solvent and can increase the selectivity of the extraction by adjusting the pressure and temperature. This method can also be used to extract other cannabinoids such as CBG and CBC. Another method of extracting cannabinoids from cannabis is to use butane or propane as a solvent. This method is known as "BHO" (butane-hash-oil) or "PHO" (propane-hash-oil) extraction. The method is effective, but also dangerous as the solvents are flammable and can cause an explosion or fire. The method is often used by do-it-yourself (DIY) cannabis producers who do not have the necessary resources or skills to use other methods. The choice of cannabinoid extraction method from cannabis depends on many factors, including the availability of resources and expertise, the size of the production batch and the desired cannabinoid profile. A method that is effective in one scenario may not necessarily be effective in another. It is also important to note that not all methods are safe, and some can be dangerous.

Making oils and tinctures from cannabis

Making oils and tinctures from cannabis is a popular method of extracting the active compounds of cannabis and using them for medicinal or recreational purposes. Cannabis contains a variety of compounds, including cannabinoids such as THC and CBD, terpenes and flavonoids, which are known for their therapeutic properties. There are various methods of producing cannabis oil and tinctures, including the use of alcohol, oil and CO2 extraction. Each method has its pros and cons and can produce different results. Alcohol extraction is one of the oldest methods of producing cannabis oil and tinctures. This method is relatively simple and requires few tools and materials. It begins with the choice of cannabis flowers to be used for the extraction. The quality of the flowers used is an important factor in the final product. Ideally, the flowers should be fresh and of high quality in order to achieve a better yield of active ingredients. Once the cannabis flowers have been selected, they are crushed and placed in a glass jar. A sufficient amount of alcohol (usually ethanol or isopropyl alcohol) is added to completely cover the flowers. The mixture is then steeped for several hours or overnight to extract the active ingredients from the flowers. After steeping, the mixture is poured through a fine sieve or coffee filter to remove the solids. The resulting liquid mixture contains the active ingredients of the cannabis and the alcohol that was used as a solvent. The mixture is then heated in a double-walled glass container to vaporize the alcohol and leave behind the pure cannabis oil. Oil extraction is another popular method of producing cannabis oil. In this method, oil is used as a solvent to extract the active ingredients of the cannabis. The choice of oil is important as it can affect the flavor and consistency of the final product. Popular oils for cannabis oil extraction are olive oil, coconut oil and hemp oil. The production of cannabis oil with oil begins with the selection of the cannabis flowers to be used. The flowers are crushed and placed in a glass jar. The oil is then added to completely cover the flowers. The mixture is steeped for several hours or overnight to extract the active ingredients from the flowers. After steeping, the mixture is poured through a fine sieve or coffee filter to remove the solids. The resulting liquid mixture contains the cannabis oil.

Production of cannabis butter and oil

Cannabis butter and oil are popular ingredients in the kitchen, especially when preparing medicinal or recreational cannabis products. Both can be made from different strains of cannabis, selected according to the desired effects. Cannabis butter and oil are made by extracting THC and other cannabinoids from cannabis with a carrier oil or butter. In this article, we will look at the production of cannabis butter and oil. Making cannabis butter: Step 1: Prepare the raw materials To make cannabis butter, you first need cannabis flowers that are rich in THC and other cannabinoids. The flowers should be well dried and de-stemmed to avoid mold growth. You can also use sugar leaves or other parts of the plant that are rich in cannabinoids. Step 2: Decarboxylation The next step in making cannabis butter is to decarboxylate the cannabis flowers. This process activates the THC and other cannabinoids in the plant and makes them bioavailable. To do this, place the cannabis flowers in a flat layer on a baking sheet and heat them at 110-120°C in the oven for 30-40 minutes. This process will activate the THC and give you the maximum potency. Step 3: Extract butter After decarboxylation, add the cannabis flowers to a stew pot with butter. You can also use oil to extract the cannabinoids. The butter and cannabis flowers should be cooked over a low heat for 2-3 hours. It is important to stir regularly to ensure that the butter does not burn. Step 4: Remove the material After you have cooked the mixture for 2-3 hours, you need to remove the material. You can do this by pouring the mixture through a sieve or filter. This will separate the butter from the cannabis flowers. Step 5: Cool and store Once you have removed the material, you need to let the cannabis butter cool before pouring it into a container. You can store it in the fridge to ensure it stays shelf-stable. Making cannabis oil: Step 6: Prepare the raw materials To make cannabis oil, you will need cannabis flowers or other parts of the plant that are rich in THC and other cannabinoids. The flowers should be well dried and de-stemmed to avoid mold growth. Step 7: Decarboxylation As with the production of cannabis butter, decarboxylation is an important step in the production of cannabis oil. The cannabis flowers should be heated in the oven at 110-120°C for 30-40 minutes. This activates the THC.

Use of cannabis in medicine

The use of cannabis in medicine has become increasingly important in recent years. More and more countries are legalizing medical cannabis for patients with certain conditions. There is a growing body of research supporting the efficacy of cannabis in the treatment of various diseases and symptoms. In this article, we will look at the use of cannabis in medicine and which conditions and symptoms may benefit from treatment with cannabis. Cannabis is a plant that contains several compounds known as cannabinoids. The two best known cannabinoids are tetrahydrocannabinol (THC) and cannabidiol (CBD). THC is responsible for the psychoactive effects of cannabis, while CBD is non-psychoactive but has some of the therapeutic properties of cannabis. Cannabis can be ingested in a variety of ways, including smoking, vaporizing, edibles or as a tincture. Cannabis has a wide range of medicinal uses. It has been shown to be helpful in the treatment of pain, nausea, muscle cramps and spasms, loss of appetite and sleep disorders. There is also evidence that cannabis can be helpful in the treatment of anxiety, depression and post-traumatic stress disorder (PTSD). In some cases, cannabis can be an effective alternative to conventional medication. For example, it can be helpful in treating pain in cancer patients who do not respond to conventional painkillers. Cannabis can also be used in the treatment of nausea and vomiting caused by chemotherapy and can help to increase appetite in people with AIDS or other serious illnesses. However, the use of cannabis in medicine is not without risks. Smoking cannabis can lead to respiratory problems and can increase the risk of lung cancer. In addition, cannabis can have psychoactive effects that can lead to anxiety, paranoia and hallucinations, especially in people with a history of mental illness. In addition, long-term use of cannabis can impair memory and concentration. It is important to emphasize that the use of cannabis in medicine should be done under medical supervision. It is also important to note that not all cannabis products are the same. The concentration of THC and CBD can vary between different products, and it is important to find the right product and dosage for the individual patient. One area where the use of cannabis in medicine shows promise is in the treatment of epilepsy. One form of medical cannabis that has been developed specifically for the treatment of epilepsy is Epidiolex. Epidiolex contains a high concentration of CBD.

Recreational use of cannabis

Cannabis is a psychoactive plant that is used recreationally by many people due to its relaxing and euphoric effects. Although it has been legalized in some countries, it is still illegal in others, leading to a debate about its use and potential risks. One reason why cannabis is used recreationally is that it has a relaxing effect.

Many people use cannabis to relieve stress or calm themselves down. It can also help to improve mood by having a euphoric effect and creating a sense of well-being. In addition, cannabis can also help to boost creativity. Many people find that using cannabis allows them to have ideas more easily and allows their thoughts to flow more freely. This can be beneficial for artists, writers and other creative people. Another reason for using cannabis recreationally is the social component. Many people enjoy using cannabis in a group and sharing it as a kind of communal experience. It can help to deepen conversations, promote laughter and simply have a good time. However, there are also potential risks associated with using cannabis recreationally. One of these is addiction. Cannabis contains THC, which is a psychoactive substance that activates the brain's reward system. With regular use, this can lead to physical and psychological dependence. Another risk is the impairment of cognitive functions. Cannabis can impair concentration, reduce memory performance and slow down reaction times. This can be particularly dangerous when using cannabis before driving a vehicle or operating machinery. Another potential danger is the use of cannabis in conjunction with other substances or medications. It can enhance or impair the effects of other substances, which can lead to unpredictable reactions. It is also important to note that the effects of cannabis can vary from person to person. Some people may develop a higher tolerance and may require larger doses to achieve the desired effect. Others may be more sensitive to the effects of cannabis and even a small amount can lead to unwanted side effects. In some countries, the recreational use of cannabis has been legalized, which has led to a debate about its pros and cons. Some argue that legalizing cannabis can help curb the black market and increase tax revenues. It could also help to facilitate access to high-quality products.

Legal cannabis industry

The legal cannabis industry is a rapidly evolving sector that has developed rapidly in many parts of the world in recent years. This industry involves the cultivation, processing and sale of cannabis products that can be used for medicinal, therapeutic or recreational purposes. In this article, we will look at the different aspects of the legal cannabis industry and discuss how it is impacting the economy and society. One of the biggest changes that the legal cannabis industry has brought about in many countries around the world is job creation. Job creation is an important factor that contributes to the economic development of a country. The cannabis industry provides many jobs in various fields such as cultivation, processing, sales and transportation. Many people have found jobs because of the legal cannabis industry, contributing to their country's economy. Another important aspect of the legal cannabis industry is the increase in tax revenue. Many governments have seen the legalization of cannabis products as a way to generate additional revenue. By taxing cannabis products, governments can generate additional revenue that they can use for various purposes. For example, they can use the money to expand infrastructure, improve the education system or support communities in need. Another positive aspect of the legal cannabis industry is the opportunity to combat the illegal market. The illegal trade in cannabis products has long been a problem in many countries around the world. By legalizing cannabis products, governments can curb the illegal market and reduce associated problems such as drug-related crime and corruption. In addition, they can ensure that cannabis products are safe and of high quality as they are monitored by regulatory authorities. Another important factor in favor of the legal cannabis industry is the ability to provide medical and therapeutic benefits. Cannabis products are used in many countries for medicinal purposes to relieve pain, reduce nausea and treat symptoms of diseases such as cancer, epilepsy and multiple sclerosis. By legalizing cannabis products, patients affected by these diseases can safely and legally access the products they need to alleviate their symptoms. However, there are also some challenges associated with the legal cannabis industry. One of these challenges is that there is still a lot of prejudice and stigma associated with cannabis. Many people still see cannabis as a dangerous drug that is addictive and can lead to mental health problems. It is important to educate people about this.

Growing cannabis as a business

The cultivation of cannabis is a lucrative industry that has grown significantly in recent years due to increasing legalization in various countries. Most countries have strict regulations on the cultivation of cannabis and only a few countries have introduced full legalization. In this article, we will focus on growing cannabis as a business and highlight the different aspects that make up a successful business. First of all, it is important to understand that growing cannabis is a complex business that requires specialized knowledge and skills. It is important to have a solid education in this field before deciding to start a business. There are special courses and training programs that are offered to acquire the necessary skills. Successful cannabis cultivation requires a lot of planning and preparation. It is important to choose the location carefully to ensure that the plants receive the optimal conditions. The location should offer sufficient space and at the same time be safe and protected. The plants need sufficient sunlight, water and nutrients to grow and thrive. It is also important to choose the right strain to achieve the desired THC content. The cost of growing cannabis can be high. It requires a significant investment in equipment, such as lighting, irrigation systems, ventilation, nutrients and security systems. Employee wages must also be considered. It is important to find a balance between the costs and the expected profit in order to build a successful business. Another important aspect of cannabis cultivation is compliance with laws and regulations. Each country has different regulations and it is important to know and comply with them. Special licenses and permits may be required to legally grow cannabis. It is important to start these processes early to avoid delays or problems. Marketing is another important factor when growing cannabis as a business. It is important to have a clear strategy to attract and retain customers. Using social media, advertising and marketing tools can help to increase awareness of your business and attract customers. It's also important to produce high-quality cannabis to build your business's reputation and retain customers. An important trend in cannabis cultivation is the transition to sustainable and organic growing methods. More and more customers prefer products that are produced in an environmentally friendly and sustainable way. The use of renewable energy, organic nutrients and water conservation are important factors in cultivation.

Risks and challenges of cannabis cultivation

Cannabis cultivation poses many risks and challenges, both for recreational and medicinal use. In many countries, the cultivation of cannabis is illegal, which brings additional risks. This article discusses some of the main challenges and risks of cannabis cultivation. Criminal consequences Growing cannabis is illegal in many countries. If you are caught growing cannabis, this can have criminal consequences. This can range from a fine to a prison sentence. In some countries, growing cannabis can even be punishable by the death penalty. Health risks Cannabis is a psychoactive substance that carries many health risks. The use of cannabis can lead to addiction and impair cognitive performance. There is also evidence that long-term use of cannabis can lead to mental illnesses such as depression, anxiety and schizophrenia. Environmental pollution Cannabis cultivation can also lead to environmental pollution. Most cannabis growers use synthetic fertilizers and pesticides to promote plant growth and fight disease. These chemicals can leach into the groundwater and pollute the environment. In addition, growing cannabis requires a lot of water and energy, which can lead to a high ecological footprint. Pests and diseases Like all plants, cannabis plants can be attacked by pests and diseases. When this happens, the yield of the crop can be significantly reduced. To prevent this, cannabis growers often have to use pesticides and fungicides, which can damage not only the plants but also the environment and people's health. Contamination Cannabis plants are susceptible to contamination by molds and other microorganisms that can occur during plant cultivation and storage. Contaminated cannabis can cause serious health problems, especially in people with a weakened immune system. Fire hazard Growing cannabis requires a significant amount of electrical energy to maintain the lighting and ventilation of the facility. This can lead to a high risk of fire, especially if the facility is not properly installed or maintained. Theft and robbery Cannabis growers are often the target of theft and robbery. As cannabis cultivation is illegal, it can be difficult to involve the police if a crime is committed. Another risk is that cannabis growers become victims of criminal organizations.

Success factors in cannabis cultivation

Note: Please be aware that cannabis cultivation is illegal in many countries. This answer is for information purposes only and is not intended as a guide to illegal activity. Cannabis cultivation has become increasingly popular in recent years as more and more countries legalize the use of medical or recreational cannabis. Success in cannabis cultivation depends on a number of factors. This article explains the most important success factors in cannabis cultivation. Genetics Genetics is an important factor in cannabis cultivation. It is important to choose the right seeds in order to achieve a high-quality harvest. There are different types of cannabis seeds that have different effects. Indica strains, for example, have a sedative effect, while sativa strains have a stimulating effect. Hybrid strains are a combination of indica and sativa and have a broader range of effects. Lighting Lighting is a crucial factor in cannabis cultivation. Cannabis needs plenty of light to grow and produce a good harvest. Special LED lamps or sodium vapor lamps can be used for indoor cultivation. The color temperature is also important when choosing lighting. Blue light promotes growth, while red light promotes flowering. Temperature and humidity Temperature and humidity are other important factors in cannabis cultivation. Cannabis prefers a temperature between 20 and 30 degrees Celsius. At higher temperatures, there is a risk of the plants drying out or being attacked by pests. High humidity can lead to mold growth, while too low humidity inhibits growth. Irrigation and fertilization Irrigation and fertilization are also crucial to the success of cannabis cultivation. Cannabis needs regular water to grow and stay healthy. However, the plants should not receive too much water, as this can lead to root rot. The choice of fertilizer is also important. There are special fertilizers for cannabis that provide the plants with all the nutrients they need. Air circulation is another important factor in cannabis cultivation.

Good air circulation prevents mold growth and promotes plant growth. It is advisable to install fans to ensure constant air circulation. The pH value is an important factor in cannabis cultivation. Cannabis prefers a pH value between 6 and 7. An incorrect pH value can inhibit plant growth and lead to deficiency symptoms. It is advisable to check the pH value regularly.

Future prospects for cannabis cultivation

Cannabis cultivation has undergone enormous development in recent years, especially in countries where the cultivation and consumption of cannabis has been legalized. The future prospects for cannabis cultivation are promising and offer a variety of opportunities and challenges. The legalization of cannabis is a trend that is continuing worldwide. More and more countries are legalizing the use of cannabis for medicinal purposes and some for recreational use. As a result, legal cannabis cultivation is becoming an important economic factor, generating considerable revenue for the state and farmers. In the future, the demand for legally produced cannabis will continue to increase as more and more people discover the benefits of cannabis. The medical use of cannabis has already proven effective in treating pain, nausea, anorexia, epilepsy, multiple sclerosis and other conditions. Future research may contribute to cannabis being used as a treatment option for even more conditions. The increasing demand for cannabis will also lead to increased production. New cultivation methods and technologies are being developed to increase the quality and yield of cannabis. Automated systems will make the cultivation of cannabis even more efficient and cost-effective. Another important factor in the future of cannabis cultivation is the increasing importance of sustainable cultivation. The environmental impact of cannabis cultivation must be reduced in order to minimize the negative effects on the environment. Various approaches are available here, such as the use of renewable energies and the use of organic fertilizers. In the future, there will also be new trends in the consumption of cannabis that will influence cultivation. For example, there could be new varieties of cannabis designed for specific effects or flavors. The way cannabis is consumed could also change. The use of vaporizers and edibles is becoming increasingly popular, which will increase the demand for high-quality cannabis. Another challenge for cannabis cultivation will be regulation. As cannabis is still illegal in many countries, there are different regulatory standards. In the future, however, there will be increasing standardization to ensure the quality and safety of cannabis products. This will also affect the cultivation of cannabis, as farmers will have to adhere to certain standards in order to sell their products. Finally, cannabis cultivation will also play an important role in job creation. Legal cannabis cultivation can be a valuable source of income for farmers and create new jobs in the industry. From the cultivation and harvesting phase to the processing and marketing of cannabis products, there are a variety of employment opportunities.

Cannabis cultivation in different countries and cultures

Cannabis cultivation is a controversial topic that is treated differently in different countries and cultures. While some countries have legalized the cultivation of cannabis for medicinal and recreational purposes, other countries remain strictly against cannabis cultivation. In this article, we will look at cannabis cultivation in different countries and cultures. United States of America The United States of America was one of the first countries to legalize the cultivation of medical cannabis. Since then, several states have also legalized the cultivation of cannabis for recreational purposes. However, the regulation of cannabis cultivation varies from state to state. Some states allow citizens to grow a limited number of cannabis plants at home, while other states do not. However, in states where cannabis cultivation is legal, cultivation must be done in accordance with local laws and regulations. The Netherlands The Netherlands is known for its liberal drug policy and the famous coffeeshop concept. Although the cultivation of cannabis is illegal in the Netherlands, there is a tolerance policy towards cannabis cultivation for personal use. This means that a limited number of cannabis plants may be grown for personal use without the threat of criminal penalties. The

Netherlands also has special cannabis cultivation clubs where members can grow cannabis together. Morocco Morocco is one of the largest countries in which cannabis is cultivated. Most cannabis plants are grown in the Rif Mountains, which are known for their mild climate and fertile soil. Although the cultivation of cannabis is illegal in Morocco, cultivation is widespread in some regions of the country and has a long history. Cannabis cultivation is an important source of income for many families in Morocco, especially in rural areas. India Cannabis has been part of the culture in India for centuries and is often used for religious and medicinal purposes. Cannabis cultivation is illegal in India, but there are many regions in the country where cannabis is grown. In some rural areas, cannabis is grown as part of traditional agriculture. Most cannabis plants in India are grown for personal use and not for commercial sale. Jamaica Jamaica is known for its reggae music, beaches and laid-back culture. Cannabis has long been part of the culture in Jamaica and is often referred to as 'ganja'. Although the cultivation of cannabis is illegal in Jamaica, the cultivation of cannabis is tolerated by the government and many Jamaicans grow cannabis for personal use. Jamaica also has a growing legal cannabis industry that is supported by foreign investors.

Environmental awareness in cannabis cultivation

The cultivation of cannabis is a topic that is often controversial in society. Some see it as a way of meeting the need for medicinal cannabis, while others reject cultivation on ethical grounds. Regardless of personal attitudes, however, there is another important component that needs to be taken into account in this topic - the environmental awareness of cannabis cultivation. Cannabis is a plant that, like any other crop, has an environmental impact. Cultivation requires water, fertilizers and energy, all of which can impact the environment in different ways. However, there are measures that can be taken to make cultivation more environmentally friendly. One of the most important measures is the use of environmentally friendly fertilizers. The use of synthetic fertilizers can affect the environment as they can cause pollution of the soil and water. Natural fertilizers such as compost or animal manure are a better option as they promote plant growth while improving soil quality. Another way to reduce the environmental footprint of cannabis cultivation is to avoid the use of pesticides or use only environmentally friendly alternatives. Pesticides can be toxic if used improperly and can affect both soil life and the ecosystem. Energy efficiency is also an important factor in cannabis cultivation. The use of artificial lighting is one of the main sources of energy consumption in indoor growing. The use of energy-efficient lighting systems, such as LED lamps, can reduce energy consumption and make cultivation more environmentally friendly. Another way to reduce energy consumption is to use natural sunlight sources when possible. If cannabis cultivation is done outdoors, this can be an effective way to reduce reliance on artificial light while reducing energy consumption. Sustainable water use is also an important factor in cannabis cultivation. Using irrigation systems that are tailored to the specific needs of the plants can help to reduce water consumption and maintain water quality. Rainwater harvesting is another way to reduce water consumption while protecting groundwater. Finally, it is important to minimize and recycle the waste generated from cannabis cultivation. This can be through the use of reusable containers for the plant material as well as the proper disposal of chemicals and fertilizers.

Social impact of cannabis cultivation

The cultivation of cannabis has various social impacts that can vary from country to country and region to region. In some countries, cannabis cultivation is illegal, while in others it has been legalized. However, regardless of whether cultivation is legal or illegal, it can have both positive and negative effects on society. One positive impact of cannabis cultivation is that it can be an important industry. In countries where cultivation has been legalized, cannabis cultivation can contribute to jobs and economic growth. Cannabis cultivation can also generate tax revenue that can be used to fund public services such as healthcare and education. Another positive aspect of cannabis cultivation is that it can contribute to medical research. Cannabis is used in medical research to treat various conditions, including pain, nausea and epilepsy. By growing cannabis, scientists can learn more about the effects of cannabis on the human body and develop new medical applications. However, there are also a number of negative effects that cannabis cultivation can bring. One of these is the criminalization of cultivation. In countries where cultivation is illegal, law enforcement agencies can prosecute cultivation as a criminal offense and impose harsh penalties on producers and dealers. This can overburden courts and prisons and damage the relationship between society and law enforcement. Another negative outcome of cannabis cultivation is that it can lead to environmental problems. Cannabis is a demanding plant that requires a lot of water and nutrients. If not managed properly, this can lead to soil and water pollution as well as the spread of pests and diseases. The cultivation of cannabis can also lead to agricultural land that could be used for food production being used to grow cannabis. Cannabis can also have an impact on health, especially for people who use cannabis. Regular use can lead to physical and psychological problems, such as problems with memory, concentration, learning and coordination. In some cases, cannabis can also cause psychotic symptoms. The use of cannabis can also impair driving ability and lead to accidents. Cannabis cultivation can also have an impact on the community in which it takes place. In some cases, the cultivation of cannabis can lead to an increase in crime, as illegally grown cannabis is often controlled by criminal organizations.

Ethics in cannabis cultivation

The cultivation of cannabis is a controversial topic that raises many ethical questions. In many countries, cannabis is illegal and its cultivation and consumption are considered morally questionable. However, there is a growing movement advocating for the legalization of cannabis and its cultivation for medicinal and recreational purposes. In this article, we will explore some of the ethical issues surrounding cannabis cultivation. Firstly, there is the question of whether it is morally acceptable to grow and consume cannabis. Some argue that the use of cannabis is unethical as it affects people's health and can lead to addiction. Others argue that there is no moral problem as long as the use of cannabis is responsible and moderate and does not lead to harm to oneself or others. Regardless of the moral evaluation of the use of cannabis, there are ethical issues surrounding the cultivation of cannabis. One of these issues is the question of the sustainability of cultivation. Cannabis is a plant that requires a lot of water and is often grown in dry regions. The intensive cultivation of cannabis can lead to water shortages and harm the environment. An ethical cultivation of cannabis should therefore focus on sustainability to minimize the environmental impact. Another ethical issue with cannabis cultivation is the use of pesticides and other chemicals. Many farmers use pesticides to protect their crops from pests and diseases. However, the use of pesticides can be harmful to the environment and people's health. Ethical cannabis cultivation should therefore ensure that no harmful pesticides or other chemicals are used and instead favor organic growing methods. Another ethical issue in cannabis cultivation is the question of working conditions for farm workers. Cannabis is often grown in low-income countries where working conditions are poor and workers are often underpaid and exploited. Ethical cannabis cultivation should ensure that working conditions for farm workers are fair and that they are adequately paid. Another ethical issue with cannabis cultivation is the impact on the local community. The cultivation of cannabis can lead to a change in the social and economic structures in a community. The cultivation of cannabis can lead to farmers abandoning their traditional crops and practices and focusing on the cultivation of cannabis in order to survive economically. An ethical cultivation of cannabis should therefore ensure that the local community is not negatively impacted and that the cultivation of cannabis does not lead to a dependency on a single crop. Finally, there is the question of the use of cannabis for medicinal purposes. Cannabis is often used for the treatment of pain, nausea and other medical conditions.

Cannabis cultivation and society

Cannabis cultivation is an issue that has received more and more attention in recent years as society increasingly grapples with the legalization of cannabis and the impact on society. The debate about whether the cultivation of cannabis should be legal affects not only those who consume this plant, but also society in general. In many countries, the cultivation of cannabis is still considered illegal. However, proponents of legalization argue that the benefits of cannabis outweigh the disadvantages. The advantages include, for example, the medicinal benefits that can provide relief from pain and other symptoms of various conditions. In addition, it is argued that the legalization of cannabis would help to reduce the illegal drug trade and combat the problems associated with it, such as violence and crime. However, the impact of cannabis cultivation on society depends on various factors, such as the type of cultivation and the size of the cultivation area. Small-scale cultivation in a private garden may have no impact on society, while large-scale cultivation in a rural area may have an impact on the environment and the local economy. In some countries where cannabis cultivation has been legalized, such as Canada and some states in the US, there are regulations and rules for cultivation to ensure that it is carried out safely and responsibly. This can include, for example, limiting the cultivation area, checking the quality of the plants and verifying compliance with safety standards. However, in countries where cannabis cultivation is illegal, there are often no controls or regulations in place, which can lead to irresponsible cultivation and environmental damage. In some countries where cannabis is grown illegally, the plant is irrigated and fertilized in an illegal manner, which can lead to pollution of water sources. In addition, the cultivation of cannabis can provide illegal organizations with money and power, which can lead to violence and crime. The impact of cannabis cultivation on society also depends on the type of cultivation. Growing cannabis indoors, for example, can lead to higher energy consumption as the plants need to be artificially lit and heated. This can lead to higher energy costs and therefore higher prices for consumers. In addition, the smell of cannabis can disturb neighbors, especially if cultivation takes place in residential areas. If the cultivation of cannabis is legalized, rules and regulations can help to have a negative impact on society.

Summary and conclusion Cannabis cultivation

is a complex process that requires both time and resources. There are many aspects to consider when growing cannabis, including choosing the right strain, soil quality, temperature and humidity conditions, light cycle and fertilization. To successfully grow cannabis, you need to understand the needs of the plant and ensure it receives the right nutrients, water and air. If you are growing indoors, you will also need to set up suitable lighting and ventilation to ensure the plants receive sufficient light and oxygen. There are various growing methods that can be used when growing cannabis. The most common methods are hydroponics, soil cultivation and aeroponics. Each method has its own advantages and disadvantages, and it is up to you to choose the method that best suits your needs and budget. An important consideration when growing cannabis is also choosing the right strain. There are many different strains of cannabis that can have different effects. Some strains are better suited for medicinal use, while others are better suited for recreational use. It is important to understand the characteristics of each strain before making a decision. When it comes to cannabis cultivation, it is important to abide by local laws and regulations. Growing cannabis is illegal in many countries, and it is important to ensure that you are not breaking any laws while growing cannabis. Overall, cannabis cultivation is a rewarding but challenging process. However, if you take the necessary steps and make the right decisions, you can grow high-quality cannabis that is suitable for medicinal or recreational use. Conclusion: Overall, it can be said that cannabis cultivation is a rewarding but demanding process that requires time, patience and resources. There are many aspects to consider when growing cannabis, including choosing the right strain, soil quality, temperature and humidity conditions, light cycle and fertilization. It is also important to comply with local laws and regulations to ensure that you are not breaking any laws while growing cannabis. However, if you take the necessary steps and make the right choices, you can grow high-quality cannabis that is suitable for medicinal or recreational use. Ultimately, cannabis cultivation is a growing and evolving market that will continue to grow as the demand for medical and recreational cannabis increases. It's important to keep up to date and learn about new developments and technology.

Guidance for beginners or novices

Growing cannabis can be a rewarding experience, both for medicinal and recreational purposes. However, growing cannabis requires a certain amount of care and expertise to achieve the best results. This beginner's guide to growing cannabis outlines the basics of growing cannabis, from seed selection to harvest. Choose your seeds Choosing the right seeds is an important first step. If you are growing medicinal cannabis, you should choose a strain that is tailored to your specific needs. If you want to grow recreational cannabis, you can look to the strains that are most popular in your region. Choose seeds from a reliable source to ensure they are of good quality. Decide on the right growing style There are several ways to grow cannabis, including indoor, outdoor and hydroponics. If you want to grow cannabis all year round, indoor growing is the best choice. However, if you have a limited budget and prefer a natural environment, you can consider outdoor growing. Hydroponics is an option for advanced growers and requires additional investment in equipment and technology. Set up your growing system Once you've decided on a growing style, it's time to set up your growing system. For indoor growing, you will need lights, ventilation systems and a suitable space to grow your cannabis. For outdoor growing, you will need suitable beds or pots and a good soil mix. For hydroponics, you will need special growing media and equipment. Pay attention to the light conditions Light is an important factor for the growth of cannabis. If you are growing indoors, make sure your plants get enough light by using special grow lights. Outdoor growing depends on natural light conditions, but you can support growth by placing your plants in sunny spots and protecting them from bad weather. Ensure the right humidity and temperature Humidity and temperature are also important factors for cannabis growth. The optimum humidity is 40-60%, while the optimum temperature is between 18 and 28 degrees Celsius. Make sure your growing environment meets these conditions. Water your plants regularly Cannabis needs regular watering to grow. Make sure that you do not give too much or too little water. Most cannabis plants need water every 2-3 days. Soil moisture should always be kept even.

Imprint:

Marie Moreno
Am Anger 3
06869 Coswig / Germany
Luna-Publishing.de